I0844560

Geneva Fern

The Autoimmune Protocol Cookbook: Nourishing Recipes to Heal and Thrive – Transforming Your Health Through Delicious AIP-Compliant Meals.

Copyright © 2023 by Geneva Fern

All rights reserved. No part of this publication may be reproduced, stored or transmitted in any form or by any means, electronic, mechanical, photocopying, recording, scanning, or otherwise without written permission from the publisher. It is illegal to copy this book, post it to a website, or distribute it by any other means without permission.

Geneva Fern asserts the moral right to be identified as the author of this work.

First edition

This book was professionally typeset on Reedsy
Find out more at reedsy.com

To those embarking on the transformative journey of reclaiming their health through the Autoimmune Protocol. In the face of uncertainty, fear not, for this cookbook is your companion in rediscovering the joy of nourishing your body. May each recipe be a testament to your strength and resilience. Embrace this healing adventure with courage, knowing that every wholesome bite is a step toward wellness. Wishing you a future filled with vitality, love, and the delicious rewards of self-care.

Contents

1.

2.

    1.

    2.

    3.

    4.

3.

    1.

    2.

4.

    1.

    2.

5.

    1.

    2.

6.

    1.

    2.

7.

    1.

    2.

8.

5.

6.

7.

13.

1.

2.

Preface

Thank you for picking up this cookbook.

Welcome to ***"The Autoimmune Protocol Cookbook,"*** a culinary adventure meant to empower you on your wellness quest. If you're reading this, you've probably begun an amazing and daring journey toward greater health. Whether you're dealing with an autoimmune ailment or simply want to make a lifestyle change, this cookbook is here to help you every step of the way.

You'll find more than simply recipes in the pages that follow; you'll find a road map to feeding your body and embracing the healing power of food. The Autoimmune Protocol (AIP) may appear to be a difficult task, but don't worry. This cookbook is your travel companion, providing not only tasty and gratifying meals, but also direction, encouragement, and a wealth of knowledge to help you understand the AIP journey.

Your health is important, and the decisions you make in the kitchen may have a big impact. We understand the difficulties you may experience, the uncertainties that come with change, and the occasional bouts of uncertainty. That is why this cookbook is about more than simply ingredients and recipes; it is about cultivating a good and caring connection with your body.

Remember that you are not alone on this road as you explore the varied assortment of recipes inside these pages, each made with love and thought. You can take charge of your health and make decisions that are in line with your body's specific requirements. Accept the wealth of nutrient-dense, entire foods given here, and make each meal a celebration of your dedication to health.

It's OK to acknowledge the difficulties, but it's also crucial to appreciate the minor wins. This cookbook demonstrates that eating healthy can be a fun experience. So, don't be afraid of the path ahead. Instead, seize the chance to nourish your body, experiment with new flavours and sensations, and rethink your relationship with food.

Finally, I want to express my deepest appreciation for selecting this cookbook as your companion. May it inspire, guide, and offer you delight in your culinary pursuits. Here's to your health, to bravely accepting change, and to relish the vivid tastes of a well-nourished existence.

With kindness and encouragement,

GENEVA   *FERN*

Chapter 1: Introduction

What is autoimmune protocol?

The Autoimmune Protocol (AIP) is a specialized version of the Paleo diet that focuses on reducing inflammation and supporting individuals with autoimmune diseases. The primary goal of AIP is to eliminate foods that may contribute to inflammation, gut irritation, and other symptoms associated with autoimmune conditions. It is designed to allow the immune system to calm down and reduce its attack on the body's tissues.

The AIP typically involves a phased approach:

1. **Elimination Phase**: This initial phase involves removing potentially inflammatory foods from the diet. Common exclusions include grains, legumes, dairy, processed sugars, processed oils, eggs, nuts, seeds, nightshades (such as tomatoes, peppers, and eggplants), and certain food additives.

2. **Reintroduction Phase**: After a period of strict elimination, some foods are systematically reintroduced to identify potential triggers for individual sensitivities. This phase helps individuals understand how specific foods affect their symptoms.

3. **Maintenance Phase**: Once the reintroduction phase is complete, individuals can settle into a maintenance phase where they continue to avoid foods that trigger symptoms while enjoying a diverse and nutrient-dense diet.

AIP emphasizes the consumption of nutrient-dense foods such as vegetables, fruits, high-quality meats, fish, and healthy fats. It also encourages lifestyle factors like stress management, adequate sleep, and regular physical activity, as these can influence autoimmune health.

Causes of Autoimmune Disorders:

1. **Genetic Factors**: Some individuals may have a genetic predisposition to autoimmune disorders. Certain genes may increase the likelihood of developing these conditions.

2. **Environmental Triggers**: Exposure to certain environmental factors, such as infections, toxins, or stress, can trigger an autoimmune response in susceptible individuals.

3. **Hormonal Factors**: Hormonal changes, especially in women, can influence the development or exacerbation of autoimmune disorders. Many autoimmune conditions are more prevalent in females.

4. **Leaky Gut Syndrome**: Some theories suggest that a "leaky gut," where the intestinal barrier becomes more permeable, may contribute to autoimmune disorders. This can allow substances to enter the bloodstream and trigger an immune response.

5. **Infections**: Certain infections have been linked to the development of autoimmune disorders. The immune system may become confused and start attacking the body's tissues after fighting off an infection.

Common Symptoms of Autoimmune Disorders:

1. **Fatigue**: Persistent and unexplained fatigue is a common symptom across many autoimmune disorders.

2. **Joint Pain and Swelling**: Inflammation in the joints can cause pain, stiffness, and swelling.

3. **Muscle Aches and Weakness**: Autoimmune disorders can lead to muscle pain and weakness, affecting mobility.

4. **Fever**: Recurrent or persistent low-grade fevers can be a symptom of an overactive immune system.

5. **Skin Issues:** Rashes, redness, or changes in skin texture are common in many autoimmune conditions.

6. **Digestive Problems**: Issues such as abdominal pain, diarrhoea, or constipation may occur, especially in conditions affecting the gastrointestinal tract.

7. **Mood and Cognitive Changes**: Some autoimmune disorders can affect mood and cognitive function, leading to symptoms like depression, anxiety, or brain fog.

8. **Hair Loss:** Alopecia, or hair loss, is a symptom seen in some autoimmune conditions.

9. **Sensitivity to Cold or Heat**: Certain autoimmune disorders can affect the body's ability to regulate temperature.

10. **Swollen Glands**: Enlarged lymph nodes may be a sign of an immune system response.

Explanation of how AIP can benefit those with autoimmune conditions:

1. **Inflammation Reduction:** AIP focuses on eliminating foods that can contribute to inflammation, such as grains, dairy, legumes, processed sugars, and nightshade vegetables. By removing these potential triggers, individuals may experience a reduction in overall inflammation, which is a key factor in autoimmune diseases.

2. **Gut Health Improvement**: AIP emphasizes the consumption of nutrient-dense, anti-inflammatory foods that support gut health. The gut plays a crucial role in the immune system, and many autoimmune conditions are associated with imbalances in gut bacteria. AIP encourages the consumption of healing foods like bone broth, fermented vegetables, and gut-friendly nutrients to promote a healthy digestive system.

3. **Identification of Food Sensitivities:** AIP involves a strict elimination phase, during which certain foods are temporarily removed from the diet. This elimination allows individuals to identify potential food sensitivities or triggers that may be exacerbating their autoimmune symptoms. After the elimination phase, foods are gradually reintroduced to pinpoint specific triggers.

4. **Nutrient Density:** AIP promotes the intake of nutrient-dense foods rich in vitamins, minerals, and antioxidants. These foods support overall health and provide the body with essential nutrients needed for optimal function. Nutrient-

dense choices include a variety of vegetables, high-quality meats, organ meats, and healthy fats.

5. **Balancing the Immune System**: AIP is designed to support a balanced immune system. By reducing inflammation and addressing potential triggers, individuals may experience a positive impact on their immune function. A well-balanced immune system is crucial for preventing the immune system from attacking healthy tissues, which is a common characteristic of autoimmune diseases.

6. **Improved Energy and Well-being:** Many people with autoimmune conditions experience fatigue and a general decline in well-being. AIP aims to address nutritional deficiencies, support energy production, and improve overall vitality. As individuals adopt a nutrient-rich and anti-inflammatory diet, they may notice increased energy levels and an improvement in their quality of life.

Chapter 2: AIP Basics

List of foods to include on AIP:

1. **Vegetables**:
   - Dark leafy greens (e.g., kale, spinach, Swiss chard)
   - Cruciferous vegetables (e.g., broccoli, cauliflower, Brussels sprouts)
   - Colorful vegetables (e.g., carrots, beets, sweet potatoes)

2. **Fruits**:
   - Berries (e.g., blueberries, strawberries)
   - Avocado
   - Coconut (fresh or unsweetened coconut products)
   - Apples and pears

3. **Meats**:
   - Grass-fed and pastured meats (beef, lamb, poultry)
   - Organ meats (liver, heart)
   - Wild-caught fish and seafood

4. **Poultry**:
   - Chicken
   - Turkey
   - Duck

5. **Seafood**:

   - Salmon

   - Mackerel

   - Sardines

   - Shellfish (e.g., shrimp, mussels)

6. **Healthy Fats**:

   - Olive oil

   - Coconut oil

   - Avocado oil

   - Ghee (clarified butter, if tolerated)

7. **Herbs and Spices**:

   - Fresh herbs (e.g., cilantro, parsley, basil)
   - AIP-friendly spices (turmeric, ginger, garlic)

8. **Fermented Foods:**

   - Sauerkraut (without additives)
   - Kimchi
   - Coconut yoghurt (homemade without additives)

9. **Bone Broth:**

   - Homemade bone broth rich in nutrients and collagen

10. **Sweeteners (in moderation):**

   - Honey
   - Maple syrup
   - Coconut sugar

11. **Non-Dairy Alternatives**:

- Coconut milk

- Coconut cream

- AIP-friendly nut or seed milk (e.g., coconut milk, tiger nut milk)

Foods to avoid on AIP:

1. **Grains**:

- Wheat, oats, barley, rye, and other gluten-containing grains
- Non-gluten grains like corn, rice, and quinoa

2. **Legumes**:

- Beans, lentils, chickpeas, and peanuts
- Soy and soy-based products

3. **Dairy**:

- All forms of dairy, including milk, cheese, yoghurt, and butter
- Some AIP followers may reintroduce certain forms of dairy later in the process, depending on individual tolerance.

4. **Nightshades**:

- Tomatoes, peppers (bell peppers, chilli peppers), eggplants, and potatoes

- Some people may reintroduce nightshades after an initial elimination phase, as tolerance varies.

5. **Eggs**:

- Eggs are often eliminated during the initial phase of AIP due to their potential to trigger immune responses. Some individuals reintroduce them later based on their tolerance.

6. **Nuts and Seeds**:

- Tree nuts and seeds can be inflammatory for some individuals
- This includes almonds, walnuts, cashews, and seeds like sunflower and sesame seeds.

7. **Processed and Refined Foods**:

- Foods with additives, preservatives, and artificial ingredients
- Refined sugars, including white sugar and high-fructose corn syrup

8. **Refined Oils:**

- Vegetable oils like soybean oil, canola oil, and sunflower oil
- Hydrogenated and partially hydrogenated oils

9. **Food Additives**:

- Artificial sweeteners, flavourings, and colourings
- Preservatives and other chemical additives

10. **Alcohol**:

- Many AIP protocols recommend avoiding alcohol, as it can contribute to inflammation and may affect the gut microbiome.

13

Chapter 3: Kitchen Essentials

Must-have tools and equipment for AIP cooking:

1. High-Quality Knife Set:

   - A good set of knives is essential for chopping and preparing a variety of AIP-friendly fruits, vegetables, and proteins.

2. Cutting Boards:

   - Invest in durable and easy-to-clean cutting boards. Consider having separate boards for raw meats and vegetables to prevent cross-contamination.

3. Food Processor:

   - A food processor is handy for quickly chopping, pureeing, or blending ingredients. It can be used for making sauces, dips, and even AIP-friendly baked goods.

4. Blender:

   - A high-quality blender is useful for making smoothies, soups, and sauces. It's particularly helpful for incorporating nutrient-dense ingredients into your diet.

5. Vegetable Spiralizer:

   - This tool allows you to create vegetable "noodles" from zucchini, sweet potatoes, or other AIP-friendly vegetables, providing a pasta alternative.

6. Mandoline Slicer:

   - A mandoline slicer helps achieve consistent and thin slices of vegetables, which can be useful for salads, casseroles, or dehydrated snacks.

7. Cast Iron Skillet or Stainless Steel Pans:

   - Non-stick pans may have coatings that are not AIP-friendly, so opt for cast iron or stainless steel alternatives for sautéing and frying.

8. Baking Sheets and Pans:

   - Choose baking sheets and pans that are free from non-stick coatings. This is essential for baking AIP-compliant treats and roasting vegetables.

9. Slow Cooker or Instant Pot:

   - These devices are great for cooking AIP meals with minimal effort. They are particularly useful for preparing stews, soups, and braised dishes.

10. Fine Mesh Strainer:

   - A fine mesh strainer is useful for separating solids from liquids, such as when making homemade bone broth or straining sauces.

11. **Storage Containers**:

- Having a variety of storage containers in different sizes will help you store and organize AIP-prepared meals and ingredients.

12. **Measuring Cups and Spoons**:

- Accurate measurements are crucial in AIP cooking, especially when experimenting with alternative ingredients. Invest in a reliable set of measuring cups and spoons.

13. **Herb and Spice Grinder:**

- Grinding fresh herbs and spices can enhance the flavour of AIP dishes. Make sure the grinder is easy to clean and free from contaminants.

Essential pantry staples for AIP recipes:

1. **Coconut Products:**
    - Coconut oil
    - Coconut milk
    - Coconut cream
    - Unsweetened shredded coconut

2. **Olive Oil:**
    - Extra virgin olive oil is a good source of healthy fats.

3. Flours and Starches:

- Coconut flour

- Arrowroot starch

- Tapioca flour

4. Herbs and Spices:

- AIP-friendly herbs and spices like thyme, rosemary, basil, oregano, and turmeric.

5. AIP-Friendly Vinegars:

- Apple cider vinegar

- Balsamic vinegar (without added sugars or additives)

6. Broths:

- Homemade bone broth or vegetable broth (without nightshades)

7. Canned Fish:

- Canned salmon

- Canned tuna (in water)

8. Sweeteners:

- AIP-approved sweeteners like raw honey and maple syrup (in moderation)

9. Coconut Aminos:

- A soy sauce substitute made from coconut sap. It adds a savoury flavour to dishes.

10. **Gelatin**:

   - Unflavored gelatin can be used in various recipes for texture.

11. **Canned Coconut Cream**:

   - A thickening agent and dairy substitute in recipes.

12. **AIP-Friendly Flavors**:

   - Garlic-infused oil (for those avoiding garlic)

   - Onion-infused oil (for those avoiding onions)

13. **Salt**:

   - High-quality sea salt or Himalayan salt for seasoning.

14. **Canned Vegetables**:

   - Canned artichoke hearts, hearts of palm, and other AIP-friendly vegetables.

15. **AIP-Friendly Baking Soda**:

   - Used in baking recipes.

16. **Ghee**:

   - Some AIP followers include ghee (clarified butter) in their diets.

Chapter 4: Breakfast

A variety of AIP-friendly breakfast recipes:

1. Sweet Potato and Apple Hash:

- Ingredients:
- 1 medium sweet potato, grated
- 1 apple, diced
- 1 tablespoon coconut oil
- Cinnamon and salt to taste

- Instructions:
1. Heat coconut oil in a skillet over medium heat.
2. Add grated sweet potato and cook until slightly crispy.
3. Add diced apple and continue cooking until both are tender.
4. Season with cinnamon and salt to taste.

2. Turkey and Vegetable Breakfast Sausage:

- Ingredients:
- 1 pound ground turkey
- 1 zucchini, grated
- 1 carrot, grated

- 1 teaspoon dried thyme

- Salt and pepper to taste

- Instructions:

1. In a bowl, mix ground turkey, grated zucchini, grated carrot, thyme, salt, and pepper.

2. Form small patties and cook in a skillet until fully cooked.

3. Coconut Berry Smoothie:

- Ingredients:

- 1 cup coconut milk

- 1/2 cup mixed berries (strawberries, blueberries, raspberries)

- 1 tablespoon collagen powder

- Ice cubes (optional)

- Instructions:

1. Blend coconut milk, mixed berries, and collagen powder until smooth.

2. Add ice cubes if desired and blend again.

4. AIP Avocado and Bacon Egg Cups:

- Ingredients:

- 2 avocados, halved and pitted

- 4 eggs

- 4 slices AIP-compliant bacon, cooked and crumbled

- Salt and pepper to taste

- **Instructions**:

1. Preheat the oven to 375°F (190°C).

2. Scoop out some avocado flesh to make room for the egg.

3. Crack an egg into each avocado half.

4. Sprinkle with crumbled bacon, salt, and pepper.

5. Bake for 15-20 minutes or until the eggs are cooked to your liking.

5. Plantain Pancakes:

- **Ingredients**:

- 2 ripe plantains, peeled and mashed

- 2 eggs

- 1/4 cup coconut flour

- 1/2 teaspoon baking soda

- Cinnamon and vanilla extract to taste

- **Instructions**:

1. In a bowl, combine mashed plantains, eggs, coconut flour, baking soda, cinnamon, and vanilla extract.

2. Mix until well combined.

3. Heat a skillet and spoon batter to form small pancakes.

4. Cook until golden brown on each side.

Options for both savoury and sweet breakfasts:

Savoury Breakfast Options:

1. **Sweet Potato Hash with Ground Turkey**:

- **Ingredients**: Sweet potatoes, ground turkey, onion, garlic, and AIP-approved herbs.

- **Instructions**: Sauté diced sweet potatoes with ground turkey, onion, and garlic until golden brown. Season with AIP-friendly herbs for a flavorful breakfast hash.

2. **AIP Breakfast Skillet**:

- **Ingredients**: Ground beef or lamb, chopped vegetables (bell peppers, zucchini, and spinach), coconut oil, and herbs.

- **Instructions**: Brown the meat in a skillet, add chopped vegetables and cook until tender. Season with AIP-approved herbs and enjoy a nutrient-dense breakfast.

3. **Coconut and Herb Scrambled Eggs**:

- **Ingredients**: Eggs, coconut milk, fresh herbs (parsley or cilantro), salt, and coconut oil.

   - **Instructions:** Whisk eggs with coconut milk and scramble in coconut oil. Add fresh herbs and season with salt for a dairy-free, flavorful breakfast.

Sweet Breakfast Options:

1. **AIP Banana Pancakes:**

- **Ingredients:** Mashed bananas, coconut flour, arrowroot flour, baking soda, and AIP-approved vanilla extract.

- **Instructions**: Mix ingredients to form a batter and cook on a skillet. Top with fresh berries and a drizzle of honey for a sweet and satisfying breakfast.

2. **Baked Cinnamon Apples**:

- **Ingredients**: Sliced apples, cinnamon, coconut oil, and a touch of honey (optional).

   - **Instructions:** Toss apple slices with cinnamon and bake until tender. Drizzle with coconut oil and honey for a naturally sweet breakfast treat.

3. AIP Blueberry Muffins:

- **Ingredients:** Coconut flour, arrowroot flour, blueberries, coconut oil, and AIP-friendly sweetener (like honey or maple syrup).

- **Instructions:** Combine ingredients to make the muffin batter, fold in blueberries, and bake until golden. Enjoy a grain-free and AIP-compliant muffin for breakfast.

Chapter 5: Lunch and Dinner

Main course recipes that adhere to AIP guidelines:

AIP Chicken and Sweet Potato Skillet

Ingredients:

- 1.5 lbs boneless, skinless chicken thighs, cut into bite-sized pieces
- 2 medium sweet potatoes, peeled and diced
- 1 onion, finely chopped
- 3 garlic cloves, minced
- 2 tablespoons coconut oil
- 1 teaspoon dried thyme
- 1 teaspoon dried rosemary
- Salt and pepper to taste

Instructions:

1. **Cook Chicken**: In a large skillet, heat coconut oil over medium heat. Add the chicken pieces and cook until browned on all sides.

2. **Add Aromatics**: Add chopped onion and minced garlic to the skillet. Sauté until the onions are translucent.

3. **Add Sweet Potatoes**: Stir in the diced sweet potatoes, thyme, rosemary, salt, and pepper. Cook for about 10-15 minutes or until the sweet potatoes are tender and the chicken is cooked through.

4. **Adjust Seasoning**: Taste and adjust the seasoning as needed. You can add more salt, pepper, or herbs according to your preference.

5. **Serve**: Once everything is cooked through and well-seasoned, remove the skillet from heat. Serve the dish hot, garnished with fresh herbs if desired.

Chapter 6: Snacks and Appetizers

Avocado and Bacon Wrapped Plantains:

Ingredients:

- 2 green plantains, peeled and sliced into 1-inch pieces

- 1 ripe avocado, sliced

- 8 slices AIP-compliant bacon

- Salt and pepper to taste (ensure it complies with AIP guidelines)

Instructions:

1. **Preheat the Oven:**

- Preheat your oven to 375°F (190°C).

2. **Prepare the Plantains**:

- Slice the peeled green plantains into 1-inch pieces. Ensure they are not too ripe to maintain a firmer texture.

3. **Wrap with Bacon:**

- Take a slice of bacon and wrap it around each plantain slice. Secure with toothpicks if needed. Repeat for all plantain slices.

4. **Bake**:

- Place the bacon-wrapped plantains on a baking sheet lined with parchment paper.

- Bake in the preheated oven for 20-25 minutes or until the bacon is crispy.

5. **Avocado Topping**:

- While the plantains are baking, slice the ripe avocado.

6. **Assemble**:

- Once the bacon-wrapped plantains are done, remove them from the oven and let them cool slightly.

- Top each plantain with a slice of avocado.

7. **Season and Serve:**

- Season with salt and pepper to taste or other AIP-compliant seasonings.

- Serve warm as a delicious and satisfying AIP-friendly snack or appetizer.

AIP Coconut Energy Bites:

Ingredients:

- 1 cup shredded coconut

- 1/2 cup AIP-compliant collagen powder

- 1/4 cup coconut oil, melted

- 2 tablespoons honey or maple syrup

- 1 teaspoon vanilla extract (make sure it's AIP-compliant)

- Pinch of sea salt

Instructions:

1. In a bowl, combine shredded coconut and collagen powder.

2. In a separate bowl, mix melted coconut oil, honey or maple syrup, vanilla extract, and a pinch of sea salt.

3. Pour the wet ingredients into the dry ingredients and stir until well combined.

4. Refrigerate the mixture for about 15-20 minutes to make it easier to handle.

5. Roll the mixture into small balls and place them on a tray or plate.

6. Refrigerate the energy bites for at least 30 minutes to firm up.

7. Once firm, transfer to an airtight container for on-the-go snacking.

Chapter 7: Soups and Stews

AIP-Friendly Chicken and Vegetable Stew

Ingredients:

- 1 pound boneless, skinless chicken thighs, diced
  - 2 tablespoons coconut oil
  - 1 onion, chopped
  - 3 cloves garlic, minced
  - 3 carrots, sliced
  - 3 celery stalks, chopped
  - 1 sweet potato, peeled and diced
  - 1 zucchini, sliced
  - 4 cups bone broth (AIP-compliant)
  - 1 teaspoon dried thyme
  - 1 teaspoon dried rosemary
  - Salt and pepper to taste (be sure it's AIP-friendly)

Instructions:

1. **Cook the Chicken**: In a large pot, heat coconut oil over medium heat. Add diced chicken thighs and cook until browned on all sides.

2. **Saute Vegetables**: Add chopped onion and minced garlic to the pot. Saute until the onion is translucent.

3. **Add Vegetables:** Add carrots, celery, sweet potato, and zucchini to the pot. Stir well to combine with the chicken and aromatics.

4. **Seasoning**: Sprinkle dried thyme and rosemary over the mixture. Season with salt and pepper to taste. Stir to evenly distribute the seasonings.

5. **Pour in Bone Broth**: Pour in the bone broth, ensuring that the ingredients are fully submerged. Bring the stew to a boil.

6. **Simmer**: Once boiling, reduce the heat to low, cover the pot, and let it simmer for about 30-40 minutes, or until the vegetables are tender and the flavours have melded.

7. **Adjust Seasoning**: Taste the stew and adjust the seasoning if necessary. Add more salt, pepper, or herbs according to your preference.

8. **Serve**: Ladle the stew into bowls and serve hot. Garnish with fresh herbs if desired.

Tips for batch cooking and freezing:

1. Plan Your Meals:

- Before starting the batch cooking process, plan your meals for the week. This helps you identify the recipes that can be easily batched and frozen.

2. Choose Freezer-Friendly Recipes:

- Opt for recipes that freeze well without compromising texture or flavour. Soups, stews, casseroles, and marinated proteins are often good choices.

3. Invest in Quality Containers:

- Use high-quality, airtight containers that are suitable for freezing. Consider using glass or BPA-free plastic containers to prevent freezer burn and maintain the freshness of your meals.

4. Label and Date:

- Clearly label each container with the name of the dish and the date it was prepared. This ensures you can keep track of what's in your freezer and helps you prioritize older meals first.

5. Portion Control:

- Divide your batch-cooked meals into individual or family-sized portions. This makes it easier to thaw and reheat only what you need, reducing waste.

6. Cool Before Freezing:

- Allow your cooked dishes to cool completely before placing them in the freezer. Rapid cooling helps maintain the quality of the food and prevents the formation of ice crystals.

7. Freeze Flat:

- When possible, freeze items flat in the container. This not only saves space but also facilitates faster and more even thawing.

8. Use Freezer Bags:

- Consider using freezer-friendly resealable bags for items like soups and sauces. Lay them flat for efficient use of space, and they can be stacked once frozen.

9. Include Reheating Instructions:

- If you're preparing meals for others or want a quick reference, include reheating instructions on the label. This can be especially useful for busy days.

10. Rotate Your Stock:

- Regularly cycle through your frozen meals, using older ones first to maintain freshness. This helps prevent items from getting lost in the freezer for extended periods.

11. Diversify Your Freezer Stock:

- Aim for a diverse selection of recipes in your freezer. This ensures you have a variety of flavours and nutrients readily available.

12. **Thaw Safely:**

- Thaw frozen meals in the refrigerator or use the defrost function on your microwave. Avoid thawing at room temperature to prevent bacterial growth.

Chapter 8: Salads and Sides

AIP Chicken and Mango Salad:

Ingredients:

- 2 cups mixed greens (spinach, arugula, and/or watercress)

- 1 cup cooked and shredded chicken breast

- 1 ripe mango, peeled and diced

- 1 cucumber, thinly sliced

- 1/4 cup fresh cilantro, chopped

- 2 tablespoons extra-virgin olive oil

- 1 tablespoon apple cider vinegar

- Salt and pepper (omit pepper for strict AIP)

Instructions:

1. In a large bowl, combine the mixed greens, shredded chicken, diced mango, cucumber slices, and chopped cilantro.

2. In a small bowl, whisk together the extra-virgin olive oil, apple cider vinegar, and a pinch of salt (and pepper if tolerated).

3. Pour the dressing over the salad and toss gently to combine.

4. Serve immediately, and enjoy this refreshing and nutrient-packed AIP-friendly salad.

Notes:

- Make sure to source high-quality, organic ingredients to align with AIP principles.

- Feel free to customize the salad with additional AIP-friendly vegetables or herbs.

- If you have specific sensitivities or restrictions, you may want to consult with a healthcare professional or a nutritionist to ensure the recipe aligns with your individual needs.

For a flavorful AIP side dish, you might consider:

AIP Roasted Sweet Potatoes with Rosemary:

Ingredients:
- 2 medium sweet potatoes, peeled and cubed
- 2 tablespoons coconut oil, melted
- 1 tablespoon fresh rosemary, chopped
- Salt to taste

Instructions:
1. Preheat the oven to 400°F (200°C).

2. In a large bowl, toss the sweet potato cubes with melted coconut oil, chopped rosemary, and a pinch of salt.

3. Spread the sweet potatoes in a single layer on a baking sheet.

4. Roast in the preheated oven for 25-30 minutes or until the sweet potatoes are tender and slightly crispy at the edges.

5. Remove from the oven and serve as a flavorful AIP-compliant side dish.

Notes:

   - Adjust the seasoning and herbs to your taste preferences, keeping in mind AIP guidelines.

   - Use this recipe as a base and experiment with other AIP-friendly root vegetables or herbs.

Creative ways to incorporate vegetables into your meals:

1. Vegetable Noodles:

   - Use a spiralizer to turn vegetables like zucchini, carrots, or sweet potatoes into noodle-like strands. These can be used as a base for pasta dishes or in stir-fries.

2. Cauliflower Rice:

- Grate or process cauliflower to create a rice-like texture. Use it as a low-carb substitute for rice in various dishes.

3. Vegetable Stuffed Proteins:

- Stuff proteins like chicken breasts or bell peppers with a mixture of finely chopped vegetables. This not only adds flavour but also enhances the nutritional content.

4. Vegetable Purees and Sauces:

- Puree vegetables like carrots, sweet potatoes, or butternut squash to create colourful sauces for pasta, meats, or as a topping for grains.

5. Hidden Veggies in Sauces:

- Finely chop or blend vegetables like mushrooms, onions, and carrots into sauces, gravies, or soups. This is an excellent way to sneak in extra nutrients.

6. Vegetable Chips:

- Make your vegetable chips by thinly slicing vegetables like beets, sweet potatoes, or kale and baking them in the oven. They make for a crunchy and nutritious snack.

7. Vegetable Wraps:

- Use large lettuce leaves or collard greens as wraps for your favourite sandwich or taco fillings. This reduces the carb content and adds a refreshing crunch.

8. Blend into Smoothies:

- Add a handful of spinach, kale, or other leafy greens to your fruit smoothies. The sweetness of the fruits can help mask the taste of the vegetables.

9. Vegetable Salsa:

- Create a colourful salsa using tomatoes, peppers, onions, and other vegetables. Use it as a topping for grilled meats, and fish, or as a dip for whole-grain chips.

10. Vegetable Kabobs:

- Skewer a variety of vegetables along with your favourite protein for grilling. The smoky flavour enhances the taste, and it's a visually appealing dish.

11. Vegetable Fritters:

- Combine grated vegetables like zucchini, carrots, and potatoes with eggs and a binder like almond flour to make fritters. Fry or bake them for a tasty and nutritious side dish.

12. **Layered Casseroles:**

- Create layered casseroles with alternating layers of vegetables and proteins. This is a great way to make a complete meal in one dish.

Chapter 9: Desserts

1. Coconut Berry Panna Cotta:

- **Ingredients**:
    - 1 can of coconut milk
    - 1 cup mixed berries (such as blueberries, raspberries, and strawberries)
    - 2 tablespoons gelatin (AIP-compliant)
    - 1/4 cup honey (optional, based on individual tolerance)
    - 1 teaspoon vanilla extract (omit for strict AIP)

Instructions:
    1. Heat the coconut milk in a saucepan over medium heat.
    2. Add the mixed berries and simmer until they are soft.
    3. Sprinkle the gelatin over the mixture and whisk until fully dissolved.
    4. Remove from heat, add honey and vanilla extract (if using), and stir well.
    5. Pour the mixture into individual moulds or ramekins and refrigerate until set.

2. Baked Cinnamon Apples:

- Ingredients:

- 4 apples, cored and sliced
- 2 tablespoons coconut oil
- 1 teaspoon cinnamon
- 1/4 teaspoon sea salt

Instructions:

1. Preheat the oven to 350°F (175°C).

2. In a bowl, toss the apple slices with melted coconut oil, cinnamon, and sea salt.

3. Spread the apple slices on a baking sheet lined with parchment paper.

4. Bake for 20-25 minutes or until the apples are tender and slightly caramelized.

3. AIP Pumpkin Pie Bites:

- Ingredients:

- 1 cup pumpkin puree
- 1/4 cup coconut flour
- 1/4 cup maple syrup (optional)
- 1 teaspoon cinnamon
- 1/2 teaspoon ground ginger
- 1/4 teaspoon ground cloves
- Pinch of salt

Instructions:

1. Preheat the oven to 350°F (175°C).

2. In a bowl, mix the pumpkin puree, coconut flour, maple syrup (if using), spices, and salt.

3. Scoop spoonfuls of the mixture onto a baking sheet lined with parchment paper.

4. Bake for 15-20 minutes or until set.

Substitutions for common baking ingredients:

1. **Flour**:
   - **Traditional:** All-purpose flour
   - **Substitution**: Coconut flour, almond flour, cassava flour, or tiger nut flour. Keep in mind that the ratios may need adjustment, as these flours absorb liquid differently.

2. **Eggs**:
   - **Traditional:** Chicken eggs
   - **Substitution:** For binding, use gelatin eggs (1 tablespoon of gelatin dissolved in 1 tablespoon of warm water, then cooled to a gel-like consistency). For leavening, try applesauce, mashed bananas, or commercial egg replacers.

3. **Dairy**:
   - **Traditional:** Milk, butter

- **Substitution:** Coconut milk, almond milk, or other non-dairy alternatives. For butter, use coconut oil or palm shortening.

4. **Sugar**:

- **Traditional**: White or brown sugar
- **Substitution**: Honey, maple syrup, coconut sugar, or mashed fruits like bananas or applesauce. Adjust the quantity to achieve the desired sweetness.

5. **Leavening Agents**:

- **Traditional:** Baking powder, baking soda
- **Substitution:** AIP-friendly baking powder (cream of tartar and baking soda), or use apple cider vinegar or lemon juice to activate baking soda.

6. **Binders**:

- **Traditional:** Gluten
- **Substitution:** Xanthan gum or guar gum for binding in gluten-free recipes. For AIP, use gelatin or chia seeds as binders.

7. **Chocolate**:

- **Traditional**: Chocolate chips
- **Substitution:** Carob chips or chopped carob for an AIP-friendly alternative.

8. **Nuts**:

- **Traditional**: Almonds, walnuts, etc.

  - **Substitution**: For AIP, use seeds like pumpkin seeds or sunflower seeds, or consider tiger nut flour for a nut-like texture.

9. **Yeast**:

  - **Traditional:** Baker's yeast

  - **Substitution:** AIP-friendly recipes often exclude yeast. Consider experimenting with alternative leavening agents or enjoy flatbreads and quick breads.

10. **Buttermilk**:

  - **Traditional:** Buttermilk

  - **Substitution:** Coconut milk or almond milk combined with vinegar or lemon juice to mimic the tangy flavour of buttermilk.

Chapter 10: Beverages

1. Bone Broth

- Ingredients:

- Grass-fed beef or pasture-raised chicken bones
- Water
- Vegetables like carrots, celery, and onion
- Fresh herbs (rosemary, thyme)
- Salt to taste

- Instructions:

1. Simmer bones, vegetables, and herbs in water for several hours.

2. Strain and season with salt.

2. Turmeric Tea

- Ingredients:

- Turmeric powder
- Ginger (fresh or ground)
- Coconut milk

- Water

- Honey (optional)

- Instructions:

1. Mix turmeric and ginger in hot water.

2. Add coconut milk and sweeten with honey if desired.

3. Ginger Mint Lemonade

- Ingredients:

- Fresh ginger slices

- Fresh mint leaves

- Lemon juice

- Water

- Ice cubes

- Instructions:

1. Steep ginger slices and mint leaves in hot water.

2. Add lemon juice and ice cubes.

4. Herbal Infusions

- Ingredients:

- AIP-friendly herbs like chamomile, peppermint, or rooibos

- Hot water

- Lemon or orange slices (optional)

- **Instructions**:

    1. Steep herbs in hot water.
    2. Garnish with citrus slices if desired.

5. Coconut Berry Smoothie

- **Ingredients**:

    - Coconut milk
    - Mixed berries (strawberries, blueberries)
    - AIP-friendly protein powder (optional)
    - Ice cubes

- **Instructions**:

    1. Blend coconut milk, berries, and protein powder until smooth.
    2. Add ice cubes for a refreshing texture.

6. Dandelion Root Coffee

- **Ingredients:**

    - Roasted dandelion root
    - Hot water
    - Coconut milk
    - Cinnamon (optional)

- **Instructions**:

    1. Brew dandelion root in hot water.

    2. Add coconut milk and a sprinkle of cinnamon.

7. Cucumber Basil Infused Water

- **Ingredients**:

    - Sliced cucumber

    - Fresh basil leaves

    - Water

    - Ice cubes

- **Instructions**:

    1. Combine cucumber slices and basil in water.

    2. Chill and serve over ice.

Tips for staying hydrated on the AIP:

1. Drink Plenty of Water:

- Water is the best and most straightforward way to stay hydrated. Aim to drink at least eight 8-ounce glasses of water a day, but individual needs may vary.

2. Herbal Teas:

- Opt for herbal teas that are AIP-friendly. Chamomile, peppermint, ginger, and rooibos are good choices. Avoid teas with added flavours or ingredients that are not AIP-compliant.

3. Coconut Water:

- Coconut water is a hydrating and electrolyte-rich beverage that fits well within the AIP guidelines. It can be a refreshing alternative to plain water.

4. Infused Water:

- Add natural flavours to your water by infusing it with slices of fruits like cucumber, lemon, lime, or berries. This can make drinking water more enjoyable.

5. Avoid Sugary Drinks:

- Steer clear of sugary sodas, sports drinks, and fruit juices, as they can contain ingredients that are not AIP-friendly. Stick to beverages without added sugars or artificial sweeteners.

6. Bone Broth:

- Incorporate homemade bone broth into your diet. It not only provides hydration but also offers essential nutrients and supports gut health.

7. **Monitor Urine Color:**

   - Pay attention to the colour of your urine. If it's light yellow or straw-coloured, you are likely well-hydrated. Dark yellow or amber urine may indicate dehydration.

8. **Eat Hydrating Foods:**

   - Consume water-rich foods, such as cucumbers, watermelon, and celery. These foods contribute to your overall fluid intake.

9. **Spread Fluid Intake Throughout the Day**:

   - Instead of drinking large amounts of water at once, spread your fluid intake throughout the day. Sip water consistently to maintain hydration.

10. **Consider Electrolytes:**

   - If you are physically active or in a hot climate, you may need additional electrolytes. Look for AIP-friendly electrolyte supplements or consume foods rich in electrolytes, such as coconut water.

11. **Be Mindful of Alcohol Consumption**:

   - If you choose to consume alcohol, do so in moderation. Alcohol can contribute to dehydration, so balance it with adequate water intake.

12. **Listen to Your Body:**

- Pay attention to your body's signals for thirst. If you feel thirsty, drink water. Thirst is a natural indicator that your body needs hydration.

Chapter 11: Meal Plans

AIP meal plans for different dietary preferences:

1. AIP Meal Plan for Vegetarians:

D*ay 1:*

- **Breakfast**: AIP Smoothie Bowl (berries, coconut milk, AIP-friendly protein powder)
- **Lunch:** Roasted Vegetable Salad with AIP-friendly Dressing
- **Dinner**: Baked Sweet Potato with Avocado and AIP-friendly Salsa

Recipe: Roasted Vegetable Salad with AIP-friendly Dressing

Ingredients:
- Assorted AIP-friendly vegetables (carrots, zucchini, bell peppers)
- Olive oil
- Salt and pepper (AIP compliant)

- Mixed greens

- AIP-friendly Dressing (olive oil, lemon juice, garlic, fresh herbs)

Instructions:

1. Preheat the oven to 400°F (200°C).

2. Toss chopped vegetables with olive oil, salt, and pepper.

3. Roast vegetables until tender and slightly caramelized.

4. In a bowl, mix the roasted vegetables with mixed greens.

5. Drizzle AIP-friendly dressing over the salad and toss before serving.

2. AIP Meal Plan for Paleo Enthusiasts:

Day 1:

- **Breakfast:** AIP Sweet Potato Hash with Ground Turkey
- **Lunch**: Grilled Chicken Salad with AIP-friendly Vinaigrette
- **Dinner**: Baked Salmon with Garlic and Lemon, Sautéed Asparagus

Recipe: AIP Sweet Potato Hash with Ground Turkey

Ingredients:

- Sweet potatoes, peeled and grated

- Ground turkey

- Onion, diced

- Garlic, minced

- AIP-friendly cooking fat (coconut oil, lard)

- Salt and herbs (AIP compliant)

Instructions:

1. In a skillet, sauté diced onion and minced garlic in AIP-friendly cooking fat until softened.

2. Add ground turkey to the skillet and cook until browned.

3. Add grated sweet potatoes to the skillet, season with salt and herbs, and cook until potatoes are tender.

4. Serve hot, optionally garnished with fresh herbs.

3. AIP Meal Plan for Seafood Lovers:

Day 1:

- **Breakfast**: AIP Smoked Salmon and Avocado Wrap (using lettuce leaves)

- **Lunch**: Shrimp and Vegetable Stir-Fry with Cauliflower Rice

- **Dinner**: Baked Cod with Lemon and Herbs, Steamed Broccoli

Recipe: Shrimp and Vegetable Stir-Fry with Cauliflower Rice

Ingredients:

- Shrimp, peeled and deveined
- Mixed vegetables (bell peppers, broccoli, carrots)
- Cauliflower, grated (for "rice")
- Coconut aminos (AIP-friendly soy sauce alternative)
- Ginger, minced
- Garlic, minced
- AIP-friendly cooking fat (coconut oil)

Instructions:

1. In a wok or skillet, heat AIP-friendly cooking fat and sauté minced ginger and garlic.

2. Add shrimp and stir-fry until they start to turn pink.

3. Add mixed vegetables and continue stir-frying until vegetables are tender.

4. Stir in grated cauliflower and coconut aminos, cooking until the "rice" is heated through.

5. Serve hot.

Chapter 12: Troubleshooting and FAQs

Common challenges faced on AIP and solutions:

1. **Limited Food Options:**

   - **Challenge**: The elimination of many foods can make it challenging to create diverse and satisfying meals.

   - **Solution**: Experiment with a variety of AIP-friendly ingredients. Explore different vegetables, fruits, and alternative sources of protein. Get creative with herbs, spices, and cooking methods to add flavour.

2. **Social Situations and Dining Out:**

   - **Challenge**: Navigating social events and restaurants while adhering to AIP can be difficult.

   - **Solution**: Plan by communicating your dietary restrictions to hosts or checking restaurant menus in advance. Offer to bring a dish to share at social gatherings, ensuring there's something AIP-friendly for you to enjoy.

3. **Time and Meal Preparation:**

   - **Challenge**: AIP may require more time in the kitchen for meal planning and preparation.

- **Solution**: Batch cooking can be a time-saving strategy. Prepare meals in advance and freeze portions for later use. Invest in kitchen tools that streamline the cooking process, such as a slow cooker or Instant Pot.

4. Cravings and Emotional Eating:

- **Challenge**: Eliminating certain foods may lead to cravings and emotional eating.

- **Solution:** Identify the root cause of cravings and find AIP-friendly alternatives. Focus on nutrient-dense foods to support overall well-being. Implement stress-reduction techniques, such as mindfulness or meditation, to address emotional eating.

5. Travel Challenges:

- **Challenge**: Maintaining AIP while travelling can be challenging due to limited food options.

- **Solution**: Plan snacks and meals, and pack AIP-friendly options for the journey. Research local grocery stores and restaurants at your destination that may offer suitable choices. Consider carrying portable AIP snacks.

6. Nutrient Deficiency Concerns:

- **Challenge**: With certain food groups restricted, there may be concerns about nutrient deficiencies.

- **Solution**: Focus on nutrient-dense foods within the allowed categories. Consider consulting with a healthcare professional or nutritionist to assess nutrient levels and discuss supplementation if necessary.

7. Social Isolation:

- **Challenge**: Adhering to a restrictive diet may lead to feelings of isolation from social events centred around food.

- **Solution**: Educate friends and family about AIP and involve them in meal planning. Seek support from online communities or local AIP groups to connect with others facing similar challenges.

8. Expense of Specialty Ingredients:

- **Challenge:** Some AIP-specific ingredients can be more expensive than conventional ones.

- **Solution**: Plan meals that use affordable AIP-friendly ingredients. Buy in bulk when possible, and explore local farmers' markets for reasonably priced produce. Focus on seasonal and sale items to manage costs.

9. Plateau or Slow Progress:

- **Challenge:** Individuals may experience a plateau or slow progress in managing their autoimmune symptoms.

- **Solution**: Reevaluate your diet and lifestyle to ensure strict adherence to AIP principles. Consider consulting with a healthcare professional to address any underlying health issues. Experiment with reintroducing eliminated foods cautiously to identify potential triggers.

Answers to frequently asked questions:

1. What is the Autoimmune Protocol (AIP)?

   - **Answer**: The Autoimmune Protocol, or AIP, is a dietary approach designed to reduce inflammation and support individuals with autoimmune conditions by eliminating potential trigger foods and emphasizing nutrient-dense, healing foods.

2. What foods are allowed on the AIP?

   - **Answer**: AIP emphasizes whole, nutrient-dense foods such as vegetables, fruits, quality meats, fish, and healthy fats. It excludes grains, dairy, legumes, processed foods, and certain nightshades.

3. Can I follow the AIP if I'm vegetarian or vegan?

   - **Answer**: While AIP is traditionally omnivorous, with a focus on animal products, it is possible to adapt it for vegetarians or vegans. This may require careful planning to ensure adequate nutrient intake.

4. How long should I follow the AIP?

   - **Answer**: The duration varies from person to person. Many start with a strict elimination phase for a few weeks to months and then gradually reintroduce foods to identify personal triggers. Some individuals may choose to maintain a modified AIP long-term.

5. Are there any alternatives for common allergens in AIP recipes?

   - **Answer**: Yes, there are various substitutions available. For example, coconut or almond flour can replace traditional flour and coconut aminos can be used instead of soy sauce.

6. Can I eat out while on the AIP?

   - **Answer**: Eating out on AIP may require some preparation and communication with the restaurant staff. Choose simple, whole-food options and ask about ingredient preparation.

7. Are there AIP-friendly sweeteners?

   - **Answer**: AIP generally restricts traditional sweeteners, but small amounts of certain sweeteners like honey or maple syrup might be used in moderation. It's essential to listen to your body's response.

8. Can I drink alcohol on the AIP?

   - **Answer**: Alcohol is generally discouraged on AIP due to its potential to disrupt gut health and contribute to inflammation. It's best to avoid it during the elimination phase and reintroduce it cautiously if desired.

9. What can I do if I'm not seeing improvements on the AIP?

   - **Answer**: It's crucial to be patient, as healing timelines vary. If you're not seeing improvements, consider consulting with a healthcare professional or a nutritionist to explore potential adjustments or underlying issues.

10. **How can I maintain the AIP while traveling?**

- **Answer**: Planning is key when travelling on AIP. Pack AIP-friendly snacks, research local grocery stores and restaurants, and communicate dietary needs with accommodations or hosts in advance.

Chapter 13: Conclusion

Congratulations on completing your journey through *"The Autoimmune Protocol Cookbook"*! As you close the pages of this cookbook, I want to leave you with a heartfelt message of encouragement and empowerment.

Starting the Autoimmune Protocol may have looked difficult at first, but you've demonstrated amazing fortitude and commitment to prioritizing your health. Remember, this isn't just a cookbook; it's a guide to reclaiming your well-being and adopting a body-nourishing lifestyle.

As you appreciate the delectable meals carefully designed, keep in mind that each item has been picked to promote your health journey. You've found the magic of nutrient-dense foods and the skill of preparing meals that not only satisfy your taste buds but also feed your body from the inside out.

Fear not your road; embrace it with the awareness that each AIP-friendly food is a step toward healing and resilience. Your body is a magnificent thing capable of regeneration, and with each nutritious mouthful, you give it the resources it requires to flourish.

Remember the significance of self-care and self-love in addition to the recipes. This cookbook is about more than simply what's on your plate; it's a reminder to listen to your body, relax when necessary, and celebrate tiny triumphs along the road.

Remember that you are not alone in your AIP journey. Your commitment to this revolutionary lifestyle demonstrates your inner power. Celebrate your success, no matter how modest, and relish in the great improvements you're bringing about in your life.

May your health improve, your soul soar, and your path is full of joy and vigour. Thank you for allowing "The Autoimmune Protocol Cookbook" to lead you down this road. Keep in mind that you're not simply cooking; you're creating a life of well-being one delicious and therapeutic meal at a time.

I wish you ongoing good health, happiness, and contentment on your path.

With deepest appreciation,

Geneva fern

www.ingramcontent.com/pod-product-compliance
Lightning Source LLC
Chambersburg PA
CBHW061018260726
48661CB00005B/2225